The Vibrant Keto Air Fryer Cookbook

The Ultimate Collection of Keto Recipes

Lydia Gorman

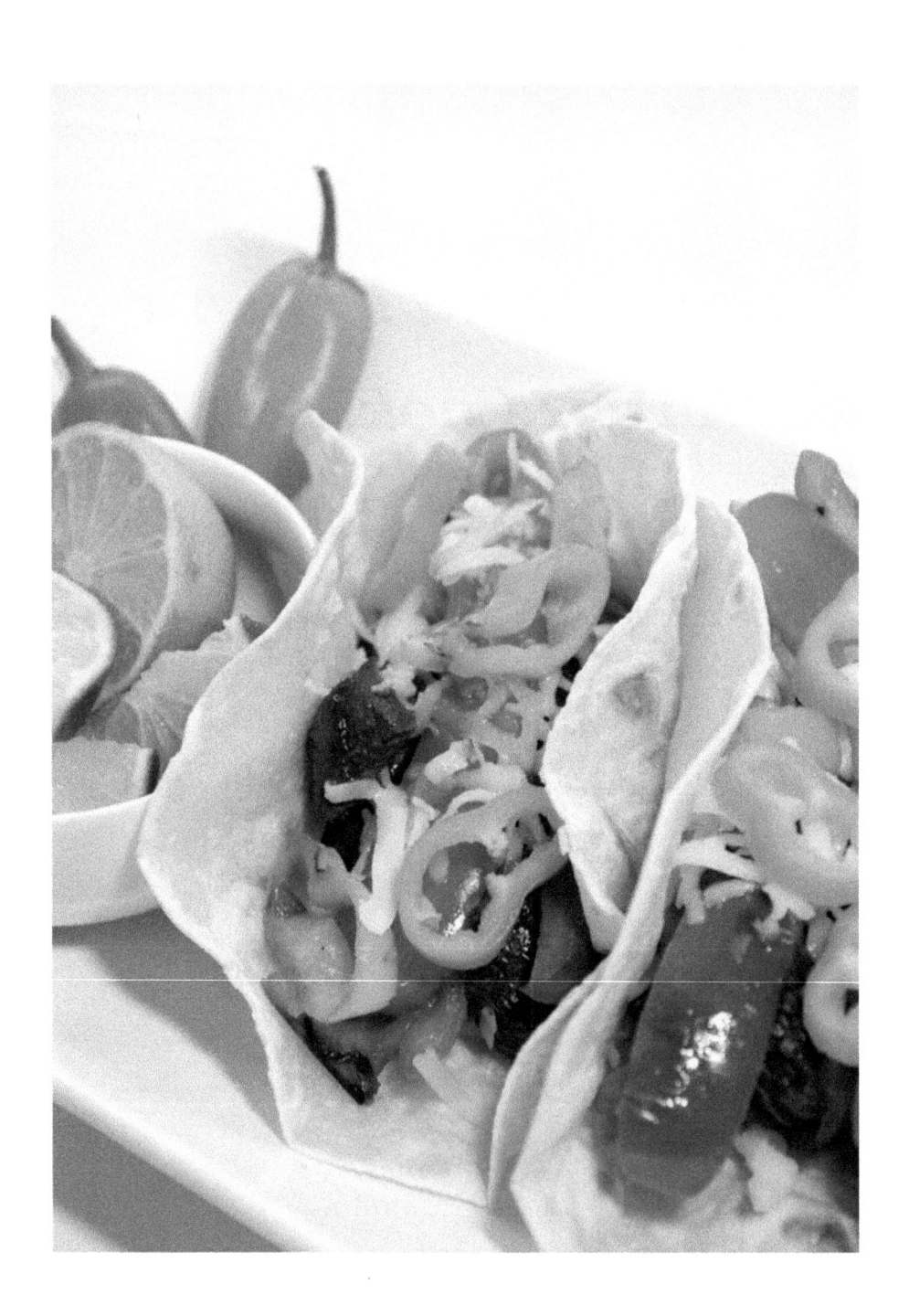

© Copyright 2020 All rights reserved.

The following Book is reproduced below with the goal of providing information that is as accurate and reliable as possible. Regardless, purchasing this Book can be seen as consent to the fact that both the publisher and the author of this book are in no way experts on the topics discussed within and that any recommendations or suggestions that are made herein are for entertainment purposes only. Professionals should be consulted as needed prior to undertaking any of the action endorsed herein.

This declaration is deemed fair and valid by both the American Bar Association and the Committee of Publishers Association and is legally binding throughout the United States.

Furthermore, the transmission, duplication, or reproduction of any of the following work including specific information will be considered an illegal act irrespective of

if it is done electronically or in print. This extends to creating a secondary or tertiary copy of the work or a recorded copy and is only allowed with the express written consent from the Publisher. All additional right reserved.

The information in the following pages is broadly considered a truthful and accurate account of facts and as such, any inattention, use, or misuse of the information in question by the reader will render any resulting actions solely under their purview. There are no scenarios in which the publisher or the original author of this work can be in any fashion deemed liable for any hardship or damages that may befall them after undertaking information described herein.

Additionally, the information in the following pages is intended only for informational purposes and should thus be thought of as universal. As befitting its nature, it is presented without assurance regarding its prolonged validity or interim quality. Trademarks that are mentioned are done without written consent and can in no way be considered an endorsement from the trademark holder.

Table of Contents

CAULIFLOWER CHICKEN CASSEROLE 9
SIMPLE BAKED CHICKEN 11
TASTY CHICKEN WINGS 14
PESTO PARMESAN CHICKEN 15
HOT CHICKEN WINGS 17
HERB WINGS 20
EASY CAJUN CHICKEN BREASTS 22
FLAVORFUL ASIAN CHICKEN THIGHS 23
BURGER PATTIES 25
ITALIAN CHICKEN 27
AIR FRY CHICKEN DRUMSTICKS 29
GARLIC RANCH CHICKEN WINGS 31
TANDOORI CHICKEN 33
RANCH CHICKEN WINGS 36
CHICKEN VEGETABLE BURGER PATTIES 38
CHICKEN SKEWERS 40
BAKED FETA DILL CHICKEN 42
PECAN MUSTARD CHICKEN TENDERS 44
EASY LEMON CHICKEN 46
WHOLE CHICKEN 47
CHEESE FAJITA CHICKEN 49
CHEESY CHICKEN CASSEROLE 52
MEATLOAF 54
CHICKEN PEPPER ZUCCHINI CASSEROLE 56

HEALTHY CHICKEN TENDERS	58
PARMESAN CHICKEN BREAST	60
SIMPLE & JUICY CHICKEN BREASTS	62
FLAVORFUL GREEK CHICKEN	64
BAKED CHICKEN THIGHS	66
ITALIAN TURKEY TENDERLOIN	68
LEMON CHICKEN BREASTS	70
MEATBALLS	72
FAJITA CHICKEN	74
ROSEMARY GARLIC CHICKEN	76
VEGGIE TURKEY BREAST	78
MUSTARD CHICKEN DRUMSTICKS	80
CHICKEN BURGERS	82
TASTY CHICKEN TENDERS	84
JERK CHICKEN	86
CHICKEN FRITTERS	88
CHICKEN NUGGETS	90
GARLIC BUTTER WINGS	92
JALAPENO MEATBALLS	94
THYME SAGE TURKEY	96
FLAVORFUL SPICED CHICKEN	98
PERSIAN KABAB	100
ASIAN CHICKEN WINGS	102
SPICY CHICKEN WINGS	104

Introduction

What's the difference between an air fryer and deep fryer? Air fryers bake food at a high temperature with a high-powered fan, while deep fryers cook food in a vat of oil that has been heated up to a specific temperature. Both cook food quickly, but an air fryer requires practically zero preheat time while a deep fryer can take upwards of 10 minutes. Air fryers also require little to no oil and deep fryers require a lot that absorb into the food. Food comes out crispy and juicy in both appliances, but don't taste the same, usually because deep fried foods are coated in batter that cook differently in an air fryer vs a deep fryer. Battered foods needs to be sprayed with oil before cooking in an air fryer to help them color and get crispy, while the hot oil soaks into the batter in a deep fryer. Flour-based batters and wet batters don't cook well in an air fryer, but they come out very well in a deep fryer.

The ketogenic diet is one such example. The diet calls for a very small number of carbs to be eaten. This means food such as rice, pasta, and other starchy vegetables like potatoes are off the menu. Even relaxed versions of the keto diet minimize carbs to a large extent and this compromises the goals of many dieters. They end up having to exert large amounts of willpower to follow the diet. This doesn't do them any favors since willpower is like a muscle. At some point, it tires and this is when the dieter goes right back to their old pattern of eating. I have personal experience with this. In terms of health benefits, the keto diet offers the most. The reduction of carbs forces your body to mobilize fat and this results in automatic fat loss and better health.

Feel free to mix and match the recipes you see in here and play around with them. Eating is supposed to be fun! Unfortunately, we've associated fun eating with unhealthy food. This doesn't have to be the case. The air fryer, combined with the Mediterranean diet, will make your mealtimes fun-filled again and full of taste. There's no grease and messy cleanups to deal with anymore. Are you excited yet?

You should be! You're about to embark on a journey full of air fried goodness!

Cauliflower Chicken Casserole

Preparation Time: 10 minutes

Cooking Time: 30 minutes

Serve: 4

Ingredients:

1 lb cooked chicken, shredded

4 oz cream cheese, softened

4 cups cauliflower florets

1/8 tsp black pepper

1/4 cup Greek yogurt

1 cup cheddar cheese, shredded

1/2 cup salsa

1/2 tsp kosher salt

Directions:

Add cauliflower florets into the baking dish and microwave for 10 minutes.

Add cream cheese and microwave for 30 seconds more.

Mix well.

Add chicken, yogurt, cheddar cheese, salsa, pepper, and salt and stir everything well.

Select Bake mode.

Set time to 20 minutes and temperature 375 F then press START.

The air fryer display will prompt you to ADD FOOD once the temperature is reached then place the baking dish in the air fryer basket.

Serve and enjoy.

Simple Baked Chicken

Breast Preparation Time: 10 minutes

Cooking Time: 25 minutes

Serve: 6

Ingredients:

6 chicken breasts, skinless & boneless

1/4 tsp pepper

1/4 tsp paprika

1 tsp Italian seasoning

2 tbsp olive oil

1/2 tsp garlic salt

Directions:

Brush chicken with oil.

Mix together Italian seasoning, garlic salt, paprika, and pepper and rub all over the chicken.

Arrange chicken breasts into the baking dish.

Cover dish with foil.

Select Bake mode.

Set time to 25 minutes and temperature 400 F then press START.

The air fryer display will prompt you to ADD FOOD once the temperature is reached then place the baking dish in the air fryer basket.

Serve and enjoy.

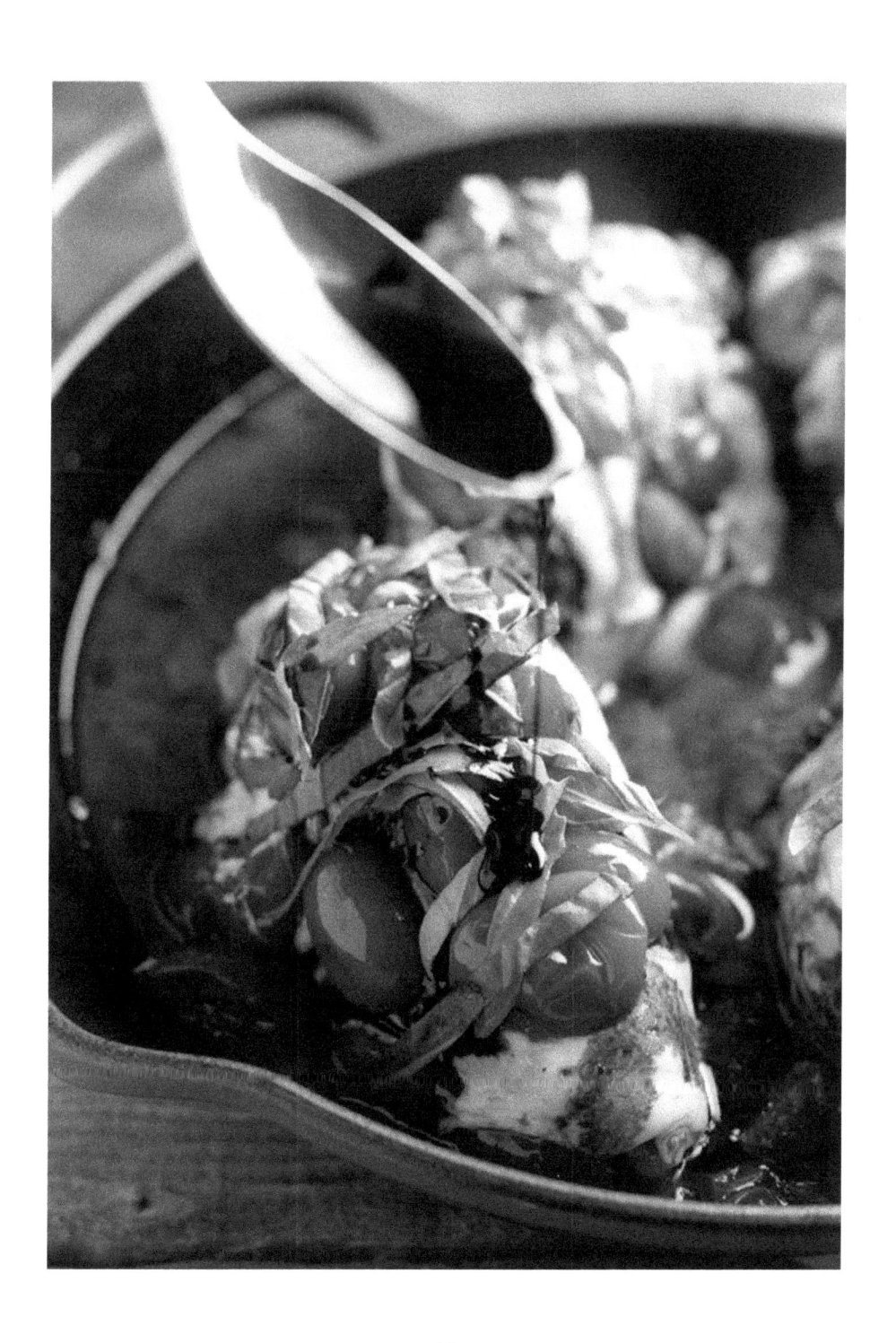

Tasty Chicken Wings

Preparation Time: 10 minutes

Cooking Time: 45 minutes

Serve: 6

Ingredients:

3 lbs chicken wings

2 tbsp olive oil

1/2 cup dry BBQ spice rub

Directions:

Brush chicken wings with olive oil and place in a large bowl.

Add BBQ spice over chicken wings and toss well.

Select Bake mode.

Set time to 45 minutes and temperature 400 F then press START.

The air fryer display will prompt you to ADD FOOD once the temperature is reached then add chicken wings in the air fryer basket. Serve and enjoy.

Pesto Parmesan Chicken

Preparation Time: 10 minutes

Cooking Time: 25 minutes

Serve: 4

Ingredients:

4 chicken breasts, skinless & boneless

1/2 cup parmesan cheese, shredded

1/2 cup basil pesto

Pepper

Salt

Directions:

Season chicken with pepper and salt and place into the baking dish.

Spread pesto on top of the chicken and sprinkle with shredded cheese.

Select Bake mode.

Set time to 25 minutes and temperature 400 F then press START.

The air fryer display will prompt you to ADD FOOD once the temperature is reached then place the baking dish in the air fryer basket.

Serve and enjoy.

Hot Chicken Wings

Preparation Time: 10 minutes

Cooking Time: 25 minutes

Serve: 4

Ingredients:

2 lbs chicken wings

1/2 tsp Worcestershire sauce

1/2 tsp Tabasco

6 tbsp butter, melted

12 oz hot sauce

Directions:

Select Air Fry mode.

Set time to 25 minutes and temperature 375 F then press START.

The air fryer display will prompt you to ADD FOOD once the temperature is reached then place chicken wings in the air fryer basket.

Meanwhile, in a bowl, mix together hot sauce, Worcestershire sauce, and butter.

Set aside.

Add chicken wings into the sauce bowl and toss well.

Serve and enjoy.

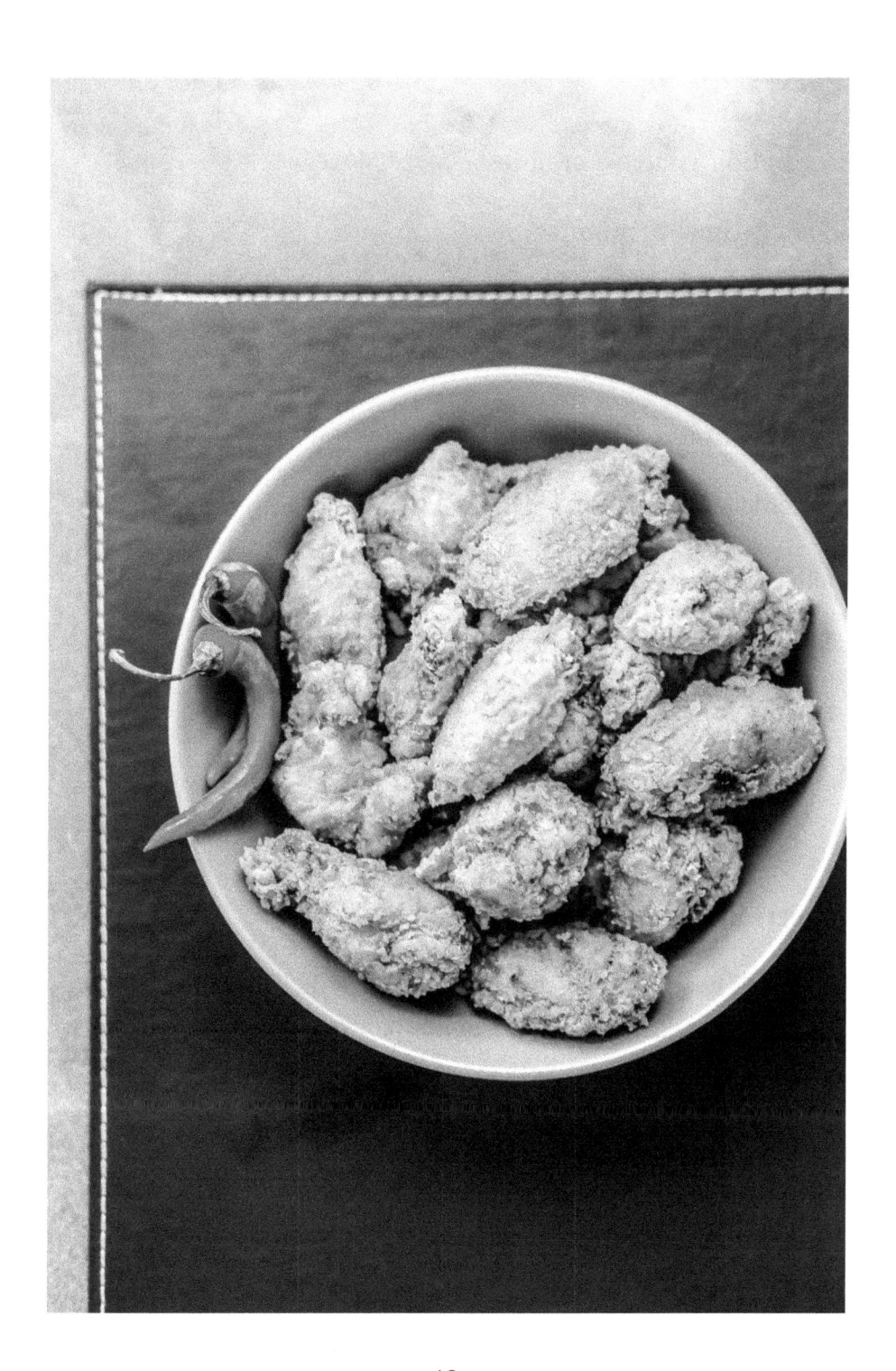

Herb Wings

Preparation Time: 10 minutes

Cooking Time: 15 minutes

Serve: 4

Ingredients:

2 lbs chicken wings

1 tsp paprika

1/2 cup parmesan cheese, grated

1 tsp herb de Provence

Salt

Directions:

In a small bowl, mix together cheese, herb de Provence, paprika, and salt.

Coat chicken wings with cheese mixture.

Select Air Fry mode.

Set time to 15 minutes and temperature 350 F then press START.

The air fryer display will prompt you to ADD FOOD once the temperature is reached then place chicken wings in the air fryer basket.

Serve and enjoy.

Easy Cajun Chicken Breasts

Preparation Time: 10 minutes

Cooking Time: 10 minutes

Serve: 2

Ingredients:

2 chicken breasts, skinless & boneless

3 tbsp Cajun spice

Directions:

Season chicken with Cajun spice.

Select Air Fry mode.

Set time to 10 minutes and temperature 350 F then press START.

The air fryer display will prompt you to ADD FOOD once the temperature is reached then place chicken in the air fryer basket.

Serve and enjoy.

Flavorful Asian Chicken Thighs

Preparation Time: 10 minutes

Cooking Time: 20 minutes

Serve: 4

Ingredients:

1 lb chicken thighs

1 tsp garlic, minced

1/2 cup water

1 tsp ginger, minced

1 tbsp sriracha sauce

2 tbsp lime juice

2 tbsp sweet chili sauce

1 tbsp soy sauce

1/4 cup creamy peanut butter

1/2 tsp salt

Directions:

In a large bowl, whisk together peanut butter, sriracha sauce, ginger, water, soy sauce, sweet chili sauce, lime juice, garlic, and salt.

Add chicken into the bowl and coat well.

Cover and place in the refrigerator overnight.

Select Air Fry mode.

Set time to 20 minutes and temperature 350 F then press START.

The air fryer display will prompt you to ADD FOOD once the temperature is reached then place the marinated chicken in the air fryer basket.

Serve and enjoy.

Burger Patties

Preparation Time: 10 minutes

Cooking Time: 22 minutes

Serve: 4

Ingredients:

1 lb ground turkey

4 oz feta cheese, crumbled

1 1/4 cup spinach, chopped

1 tsp Italian seasoning

1 tbsp olive oil

1 tbsp garlic paste

Pepper

Salt

Directions:

Add all ingredients into the mixing bowl and mix until well combined.

Make 4 equal shapes of patties from the mixture.

Select Air Fry mode.

Set time to 22 minutes and temperature 390 F then press START.

The air fryer display will prompt you to ADD FOOD once the temperature is reached then place chicken patties in the air fryer basket.

Turn patties halfway through.

Serve and enjoy.

Italian Chicken

Preparation Time: 10 minutes

Cooking Time: 25 minutes

Serve: 4

Ingredients:

4 chicken breasts, skinless & boneless

1 tbsp olive oil

For rub:

1 tsp oregano

1 tsp thyme

1 tsp parsley

1 tsp onion powder

1 tsp basil

Pepper

Salt

Directions:

Brush chicken breast with oil.

In a small bowl, mix together all rub ingredients and rub all over chicken breasts.

Select Air Fry mode.

Set time to 25 minutes and temperature 390 F then press START.

The air fryer display will prompt you to ADD FOOD once the temperature is reached then place chicken in the air fryer basket.

Turn chicken halfway through. Serve and enjoy

Air Fry Chicken Drumsticks

Preparation Time: 10 minutes

Cooking Time: 25 minutes

Serve: 5

Ingredients:

5 chicken drumsticks

1/4 tsp paprika

1/2 tsp garlic powder

2 tbsp olive oil

1/2 cup BBQ sauce, sugar-free

1/4 tsp onion powder

Pepper

Salt

Directions:

In a bowl, add chicken drumsticks, onion powder, garlic powder, olive oil, paprika, pepper, and salt and toss well.

Select Air Fry mode.

Set time to 15 minutes and temperature 390 F then press START.

The air fryer display will prompt you to ADD FOOD once the temperature is reached then place chicken drumsticks in the air fryer basket.

Turn chicken drumsticks and air fry for 5 minutes more.

Brush chicken drumsticks with BBQ sauce air fry for 5 minutes more.

Serve and enjoy.

Garlic Ranch Chicken Wings

Preparation Time: 10 minutes

Cooking Time: 25 minutes

Serve: 2

Ingredients:

1 lb chicken wings

1 1/2 tbsp ranch seasoning

3 garlic cloves, minced

2 tbsp butter, melted

Directions:

In a bowl, mix together butter, garlic, and ranch seasoning.

Add chicken wings and toss to coat.

Cover bowl and place in the refrigerator overnight.

Select Air Fry mode.

Set time to 25 minutes and temperature 360 F then press START.

The air fryer display will prompt you to ADD FOOD once the temperature is reached then add chicken wings in the air fryer basket.

Serve and enjoy.

Tandoori Chicken

Preparation Time: 10 minutes

Cooking Time: 15 minutes

Serve: 4

Ingredients:

4 chicken drumsticks

For marinade:

1/2 tsp garam masala

1/2 tsp ground turmeric

1 tsp chili powder

1 tbsp ginger garlic paste

1 tbsp fresh lime juice

1 tsp ground cumin

1/4 cup yogurt

1 tsp salt

Directions:

In a bowl, mix together all marinade ingredients until well combined.

Add chicken in marinade and mix until well coated.

Cover and place in the refrigerator overnight.

Select Air Fry mode.

Set time to 10 minutes and temperature 360 F then press START.

The air fryer display will prompt you to ADD FOOD once the temperature is reached then place chicken in the air fryer basket.

Turn chicken halfway through and cook for 5 minutes more.

Serve and enjoy.

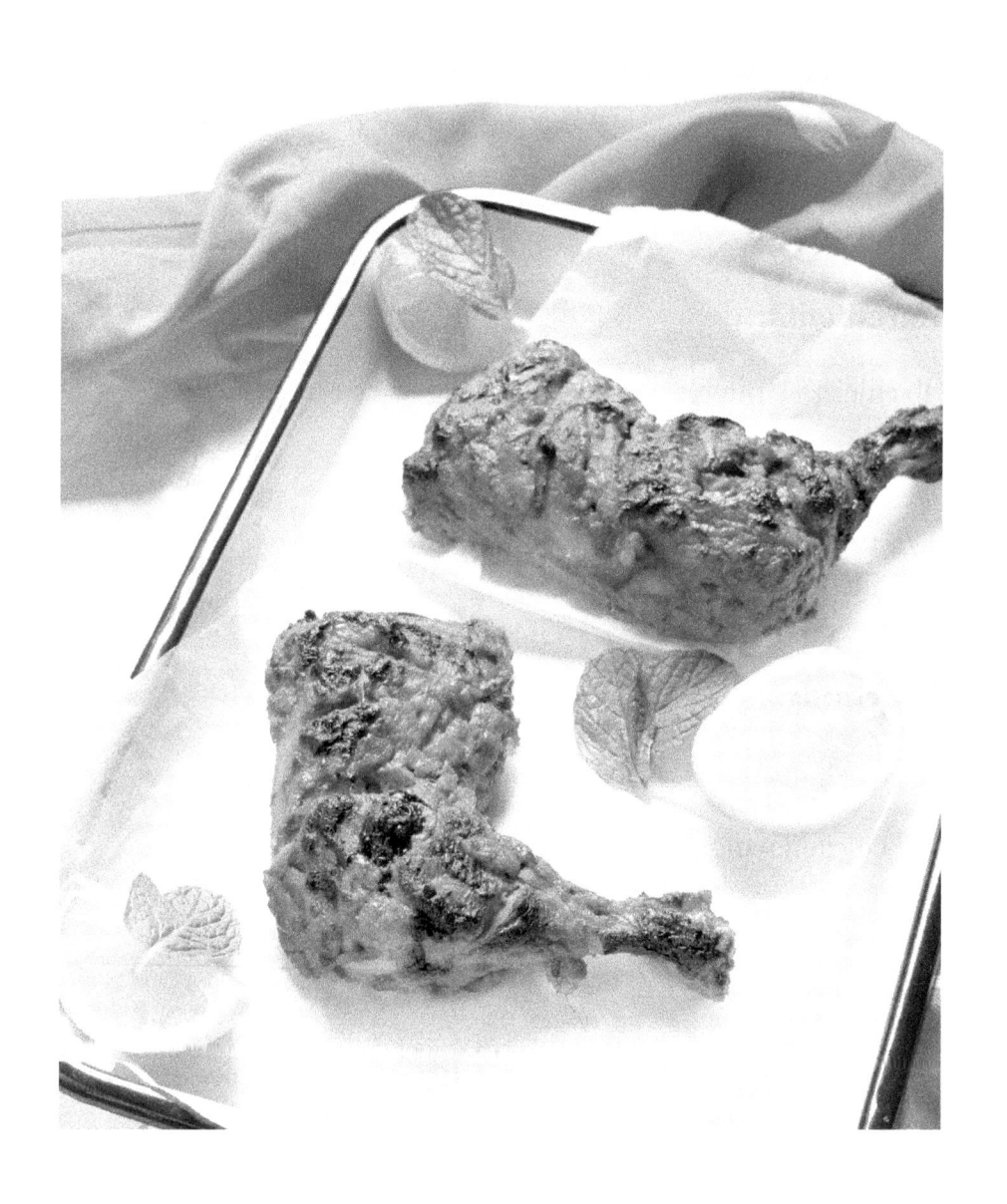

Ranch Chicken Wings

Preparation Time: 10 minutes

Cooking Time: 20 minutes

Serve: 2

Ingredients:

1 lb chicken wings

2 tbsp butter, melted

1 1/2 tbsp ranch seasoning

Directions:

In a bowl, mix together butter, and ranch seasoning.

Add chicken wings and toss well.

Cover and place in the refrigerator for 1 hour.

Select Air Fry mode.

Set time to 20 minutes and temperature 360 F then press START.

The air fryer display will prompt you to ADD FOOD once the temperature is reached then place chicken wings in the air fryer basket.

Serve and enjoy.

Chicken Vegetable Burger Patties

Preparation Time: 10 minutes

Cooking Time: 25 minutes

Serve: 4

Ingredients:

1 lb ground chicken

3/4 cup almond flour

1 egg, lightly beaten

1 cup Monterey jack cheese, grated

1 cup carrot, grated

1 cup cauliflower, grated

1/8 tsp red pepper flakes

2 garlic cloves, minced

1/2 cup onion, minced

Pepper

Salt

Directions:

Add all ingredients into the mixing bowl and mix until well combined.

Make small patties from the mixture.

Select Bake mode.

Set time to 25 minutes and temperature 400 F then press START.

The air fryer display will prompt you to ADD FOOD once the temperature is reached then place chicken patties in the air fryer basket.

Serve and enjoy.

Chicken Skewers

Preparation Time: 10 minutes

Cooking Time: 20 minutes

Serve: 4

Ingredients:

1 1/2 lbs chicken breast, cut into 1-inch cubes

For marinade:

2 tbsp dried oregano

1/4 cup fresh mint leaves

5 garlic cloves

1/2 cup lemon juice

1/4 tsp cayenne

1 tbsp red wine vinegar

1/2 cup low-fat yogurt

2 tbsp fresh rosemary, chopped

1 cup olive oil

Pepper

Salt

Directions:

Add all marinade ingredients into the blender and blend until smooth.

Pour marinade in a large bowl.

Add chicken to the bowl and coat well, cover and place in the refrigerator for 1 hour.

Remove marinated chicken from the refrigerator and slide onto the skewers.

Select Bake mode. Set time to 20 minutes and temperature 400 F then press START.

The air fryer display will prompt you to ADD FOOD once the temperature is reached then place chicken skewers in the air fryer basket.

Serve and enjoy.

Baked Feta Dill Chicken

Preparation Time: 10 minutes

Cooking Time: 35 minutes

Serve: 4

Ingredients:

2lbs chicken tenders

2 tbsp olive oil

3 dill sprigs

1 large zucchini

1 cup grape tomatoes

For topping:

1 tbsp fresh lemon juice

1 tbsp fresh dill, chopped

2 tbsp feta cheese, crumbled

1 tbsp olive oil

Directions:

Drizzle the olive oil on a baking dish then place chicken, zucchini, dill, and tomatoes in the dish.

Season with salt.

Select Bake mode.

Set time to 30 minutes and temperature 400 F then press START.

The air fryer display will prompt you to ADD FOOD once the temperature is reached then place the baking dish in the air fryer basket.

Meanwhile, in a small bowl, stir together all topping ingredients.

Sprinkle topping mixture on top of the chicken and Serve.

Pecan Mustard Chicken Tenders

Preparation Time: 10 minutes

Cooking Time: 12 minutes

Serve: 4

Ingredients:

1 lb chicken tenders

1 egg, lightly beaten

1/2 tsp paprika

1 cup pecans, crushed

1/4 cup ground mustard

1 tsp pepper

1 tsp salt

Directions:

Add chicken into the large bowl.

Season with paprika, pepper, and salt.

Add mustard mix well.

In another bowl, add egg and whisk well.

In a shallow dish, add crushed pecans.

Dip chicken into the egg then coats with crushed pecans.

Select Air Fry mode.

Set time to 12 minutes and temperature 350 F then press START.

The air fryer display will prompt you to ADD FOOD once the temperature is reached then place coated chicken tenders in the air fryer basket.

Serve and enjoy.

Easy Lemon Chicken

Preparation Time: 10 minutes

Cooking Time: 20 minutes

Serve: 4

Ingredients:

4 chicken breasts, skinless and boneless

1 preserved lemon

1 tbsp olive oil

Directions:

Add all ingredients into the bowl and mix well.

Set aside for 10 minutes.

Select Air Fry mode.

Set time to 20 minutes and temperature 400 F then press START.

The air fryer display will prompt you to ADD FOOD once the temperature is reached then place chicken in the air fryer basket. Serve and enjoy.

Whole Chicken

Preparation Time: 10 minutes

Cooking Time: 35 minutes

Serve: 4

Ingredients:

4 lbs whole chicken, cut into pieces

2 tsp ground sumac

4 garlic cloves, minced

2 tbsp olive oil

1 tsp lemon zest

2 tsp kosher salt

Directions:

Rub chicken with oil, sumac, lemon zest, and salt.

Marinate in the refrigerator for 3 hours.

Select Air Fry mode.

Set time to 35 minutes and temperature 350 F then press START.

The air fryer display will prompt you to ADD FOOD once the temperature is reached then place the marinated chicken in the air fryer basket.

Serve and enjoy.

Cheese Fajita Chicken

Preparation Time: 10 minutes

Cooking Time: 15 minutes

Serve: 4

Ingredients:

4 chicken breasts, make horizontal cuts on each piece

1 bell pepper, sliced

2 tbsp fajita seasoning

2 tbsp olive oil

1/2 cup cheddar cheese, shredded

1 onion, sliced

Directions:

Rub oil and seasoning all over the chicken breast.

Add chicken, bell pepper, and onion into the baking dish.

Select Air Fry mode.

Set time to 10 minutes and temperature 380 F then press START.

The air fryer display will prompt you to ADD FOOD once the temperature is reached then place the baking dish in the air fryer basket.

Sprinkle cheese on top of the chicken and cook for 5 minutes more.

Serve and enjoy.

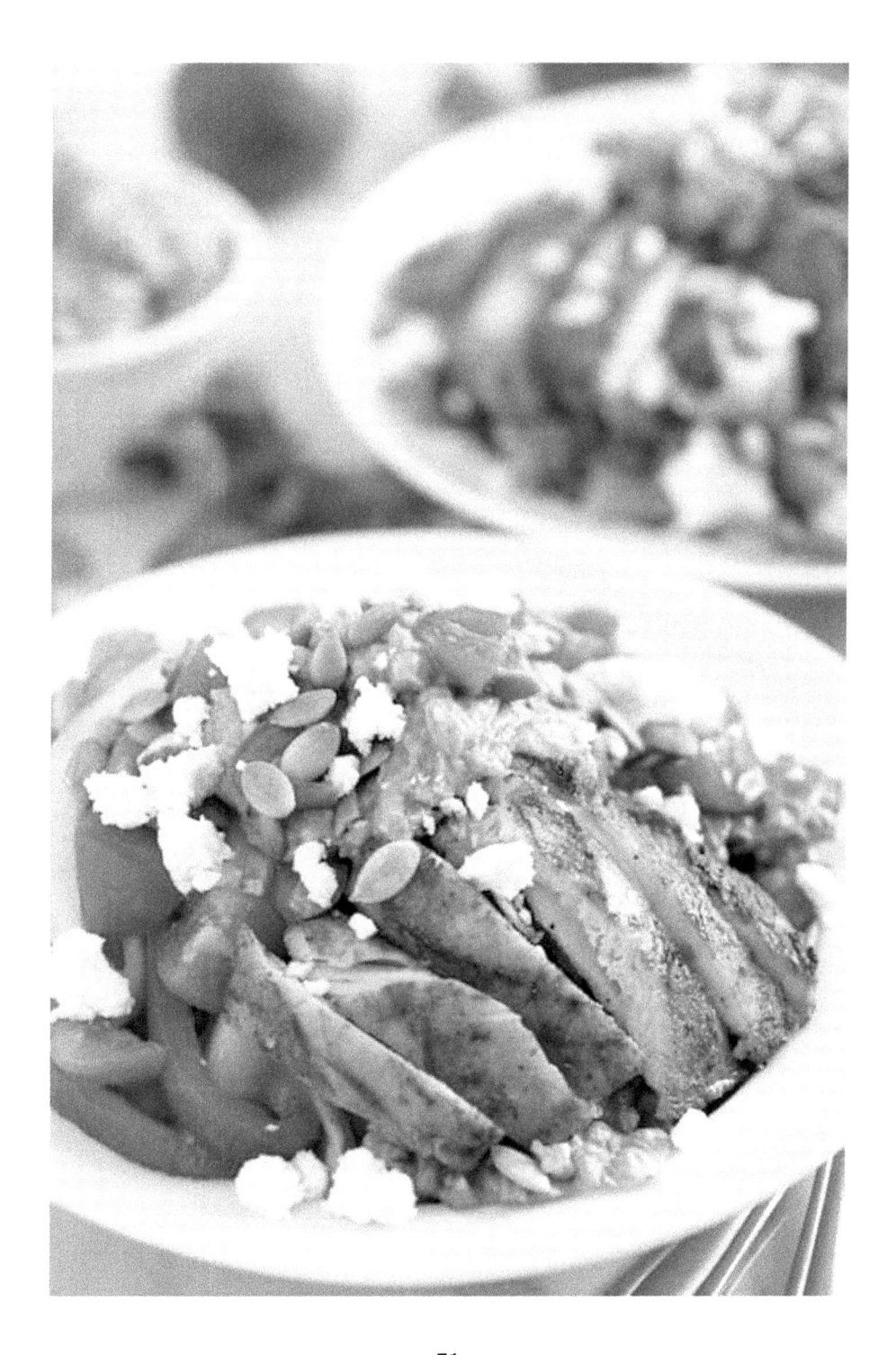

Cheesy Chicken Casserole

Preparation Time: 10 minutes

Cooking Time: 40 minutes

Serve: 8

Ingredients:

2 lbs cooked chicken, shredded

6 oz cream cheese, softened

4 oz butter, melted

6 oz ham, cut into small pieces

5 oz Swiss cheese

1 oz fresh lemon juice

1 tbsp Dijon mustard

1/2 tsp salt

Directions:

Arrange chicken in the bottom of the baking dish then layer ham pieces on top.

Add butter, lemon juice, mustard, cream cheese, and salt into the blender and blend until a thick sauce.

Spread sauce over top of chicken and ham mixture in the baking dish.

Arrange cheese slices on top of sauce.

Select Bake mode.

Set time to 40 minutes and temperature 350 F then press START.

The air fryer display will prompt you to ADD FOOD once the temperature is reached then place the baking dish in the air fryer basket.

Serve and enjoy.

Meatloaf

Preparation Time: 10 minutes

Cooking Time: 40 minutes

Serve: 8

Ingredients:

2 eggs

1/2 cup parmesan cheese, grated

1/2 cup marinara sauce, without sugar

1 cup cottage cheese

1 lb mozzarella cheese, cut into cubes

2 lbs ground turkey

2 tsp Italian seasoning

1/4 cup basil pesto

1 tsp salt

Directions:

Add all ingredients into the large bowl and mix until well combined.

Transfer bowl mixture into the loaf pan.

Select Bake mode.

Set time to 40 minutes and temperature 400 F then press START.

The air fryer display will prompt you to ADD FOOD once the temperature is reached then place the coated loaf pan in the air fryer basket.

Serve and enjoy.

Chicken Pepper Zucchini Casserole

Preparation Time: 10 minutes

Cooking Time: 40 minutes

Serve: 8

Ingredients:

2 1/2 lbs chicken breasts, boneless and cubed

12 oz roasted red peppers, drained and chopped

10 garlic cloves

2/3 cup mayonnaise

5 zucchini, cut into cubes

1 tsp xanthan gum

1 tbsp tomato paste

5 oz coconut cream

1 tsp salt

Directions:

Add zucchini and chicken to a casserole dish.

Select Bake mode.

Set time to 25 minutes and temperature 400 F then press START.

The air fryer display will prompt you to ADD FOOD once the temperature is reached then place a casserole dish in the air fryer basket.

Stir well and cook for 10 minutes more.

Meanwhile, in a bowl, stir together the remaining ingredients.

Pour bowl mixture over chicken mixture and broil for 5 minutes.

Serve and enjoy.

Healthy Chicken Tenders

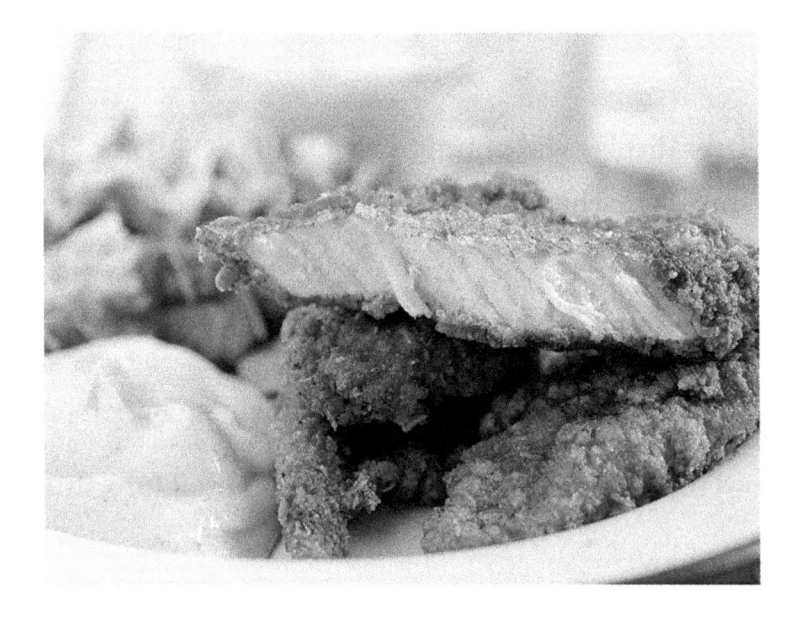

Preparation Time: 10 minutes

Cooking Time: 10 minutes

Serve: 3

Ingredients:

1 egg

1 lb chicken breast, boneless & cut into strips

1 tsp garlic powder

2 tsp Italian seasoning

1/3 cup pecans, chopped

2/3 cup almond flour

1 tbsp water

1/2 tsp sea salt

Directions:

In a small bowl, whisk together egg and 1 tablespoon of water.

In a shallow bowl, mix together almond flour, pecans, Italian seasoning, garlic powder, and salt.

Dip each chicken strip in egg then coat with almond flour mixture.

Place the cooking tray in the air fryer basket.

Select Air Fry mode.

Set time to 10 minutes and temperature 350 F then press START.

The air fryer display will prompt you to ADD FOOD once the temperature is reached then place coated chicken strips in the air fryer basket.

Turn chicken strips halfway through.

Serve and enjoy.

Parmesan Chicken Breast

Preparation Time: 10 minutes

Cooking Time: 14 minutes

Serve: 4

Ingredients:

2 eggs, lightly beaten

1 lb chicken breast, skinless & boneless

1 cup parmesan cheese, grated

1/2 cup almond flour

1/2 tsp garlic powder

1 tsp Italian seasoning

Pepper

Salt

Directions:

In a shallow bowl, add eggs and whisk well.

In a separate shallow dish, mix together parmesan cheese, Italian seasoning, garlic powder, almond flour, pepper, and salt.

Dip chicken breast into the egg mixture and coat with parmesan cheese mixture.

Place the cooking tray in the air fryer basket.

Select Air Fry mode.

Set time to 14 minutes and temperature 360 F then press START.

The air fryer display will prompt you to ADD FOOD once the temperature is reached then place coated chicken breasts in the air fryer basket.

Serve and enjoy.

Simple & Juicy Chicken Breasts

Preparation Time: 10 minutes

Cooking Time: 30 minutes

Serve: 2

Ingredients:

2 chicken breasts, skinless & boneless

1/2 tsp garlic powder

1 tbsp olive oil

1/4 tsp pepper

1/2 tsp salt

Directions:

Brush chicken breasts with oil and season with garlic powder, pepper, and salt.

Place the cooking tray in the air fryer basket.

Select Air Fry mode.

Set time to 30 minutes and temperature 360 F then press START.

The air fryer display will prompt you to ADD FOOD once the temperature is reached then place chicken breasts in the air fryer basket.

Turn chicken after 20 minutes.

Serve and enjoy

Flavorful Greek Chicken

Preparation Time: 10 minutes

Cooking Time: 30 minutes

Serve: 4

Ingredients:

1 lb chicken breasts, skinless & boneless

For marinade:

1 tsp onion powder

1/4 tsp basil

1/4 tsp oregano

3 garlic cloves, minced

1 tbsp lemon juice

3 tbsp olive oil

1/2 tsp dill

1/4 tsp pepper

1/2 tsp

salt

Directions:

Add all marinade ingredients into the bowl and mix well.

Add chicken into the marinade and coat well.

Cover and place in the refrigerator overnight.

Arrange marinated chicken into the baking dish.

Cover dish with foil.

Select Bake mode.

Set time to 30 minutes and temperature 400 F then press START.

The air fryer display will prompt you to ADD FOOD once the temperature is reached then place baking dish in the air fryer basket.

Serve and enjoy.

Baked Chicken Thighs

Preparation Time: 10 minutes

Cooking Time: 35 minutes

Serve: 6

Ingredients:

6 chicken thighs

2 tsp poultry seasoning

2 tbsp olive oil

Pepper

Salt

Directions:

Brush chicken with oil and rub with poultry seasoning, pepper, and salt.

Arrange chicken into the baking dish.

Cover dish with foil.

Select Bake mode.

Set time to 35 minutes and temperature 400 F then press START.

The air fryer display will prompt you to ADD FOOD once the temperature is reached then place the baking dish in the air fryer basket.

Serve and enjoy.

Italian Turkey Tenderloin

Preparation Time: 10 minutes

Cooking Time: 45 minutes

Serve: 4

Ingredients:

1 1/2 lbs turkey breast tenderloin

1/2 tbsp olive oil

1 tsp Italian seasoning

1/4 tsp pepper

1/2 tsp salt

Directions:

Brush turkey tenderloin with olive oil and rub with Italian seasoning, pepper, and salt.

Select Bake mode.

Set time to 45 minutes and temperature 390 F then press START.

The air fryer display will prompt you to ADD FOOD once the temperature is reached then place turkey tenderloin in the air fryer basket.

Serve and enjoy.

Lemon Chicken Breasts

Preparation Time: 10 minutes

Cooking Time: 30 minutes

Serve: 4

Ingredients:

4 chicken breasts, skinless and boneless

4 tsp butter, sliced

1/2 tsp paprika

1 tsp garlic powder

1 tsp lemon pepper seasoning

4 tsp lemon juice

Pepper

Salt

Directions:

Season chicken with pepper and salt and place into the baking dish.

Pour lemon juice over chicken.

Mix together paprika, garlic powder, and lemon pepper seasoning and sprinkle over chicken.

Add butter slices on top of the chicken.

Select Bake mode.

Set time to 30 minutes and temperature 350 F then press START.

The air fryer display will prompt you to ADD FOOD once the temperature is reached then place the baking dish in the air fryer basket.

Serve and enjoy.

Meatballs

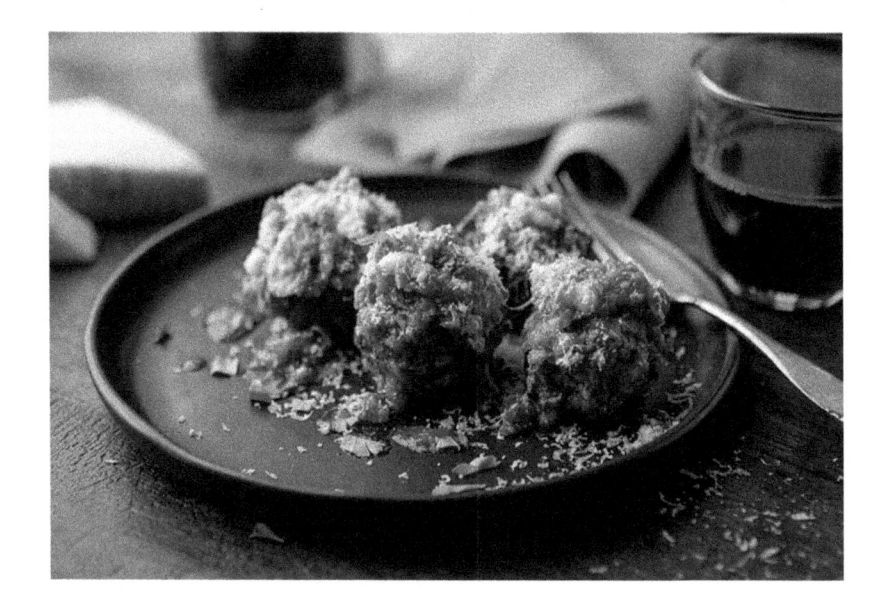

Preparation Time: 10 minutes

Cooking Time: 20 minutes

Serve: 6

Ingredients:

1 lb ground turkey

1 tbsp basil, chopped

1/3 cup coconut flour

2 cups zucchini, grated

1 tbsp dried onion flakes

2 eggs, lightly beaten

1 tbsp nutritional yeast

1 tsp dried oregano

1 tbsp garlic, minced

1 tsp cumin

Pepper

Salt

Directions:

Add all ingredients into the bowl and mix until just combined.

Make small balls from the meat mixture.

Select Bake mode.

Set time to 20 minutes and temperature 400 F then press START.

The air fryer display will prompt you to ADD FOOD once the temperature is reached then place meatballs in the air fryer basket.

Serve and enjoy.

Fajita Chicken

Preparation Time: 10 minutes

Cooking Time: 15 minutes

Serve: 4

Ingredients:

4 chicken breasts, make horizontal cuts on each piece

2 tbsp fajita seasoning

2 tbsp olive oil

1 onion, sliced

1 bell pepper, sliced

Directions:

Brush chicken with oil and season with fajita seasoning.

Select Bake mode.

Set time to 15 minutes and temperature 375 F then press START.

The air fryer display will prompt you to ADD FOOD once the temperature is reached then add chicken, onion, and bell pepper in the air fryer basket.

Serve and enjoy.

Rosemary Garlic Chicken

Preparation Time: 10 minutes

Cooking Time: 25 minutes

Serve: 4

Ingredients:

1 lb chicken breasts, skinless, boneless, and cubed

2 tbsp chives, chopped

1 tbsp fresh lemon juice

1 tsp garlic powder

1 tbsp rosemary, chopped

1 tbsp garlic, minced

2 tbsp olive oil

Pepper

Salt

Directions:

Add all ingredients into the bowl and toss well.

Select Air Fry mode.

Set time to 25 minutes and temperature 370 F then press START.

The air fryer display will prompt you to ADD FOOD once the temperature is reached then add the chicken mixture in the air fryer basket.

Serve and enjoy.

Veggie Turkey Breast

Preparation Time: 10 minutes

Cooking Time: 45 minutes

Serve: 4

Ingredients:

1lb turkey breast, cut into 1-inch cubes

1 cup mushrooms, cleaned

1/2 lb Brussels sprouts, cut in half

1 tsp garlic powder

2 tbsp olive oil

Pepper

Salt

Directions:

In a small bowl, mix oil, garlic powder, pepper, and salt.

In a baking dish, mix together turkey, mushrooms, and Brussels sprouts.

Pour oil mixture on top.

Cover dish with foil.

Select Bake mode.

Set time to 45 minutes and temperature 350 F then press START.

The air fryer display will prompt you to ADD FOOD once the temperature is reached then place the baking dish in the air fryer basket.

Serve and enjoy.

Mustard Chicken Drumsticks

Preparation Time: 10 minutes

Cooking Time: 12 minutes

Serve: 2

Ingredients:

2 chicken drumsticks

1/2 tsp ginger garlic paste

1/2 tsp mustard

1/2 tbsp olive oil

Pepper

Salt

Directions:

Add chicken wings into the bowl.

Add remaining ingredients and toss well.

Select Air Fry mode.

Set time to 12 minutes and temperature 350 F then press START.

The air fryer display will prompt you to ADD FOOD once the temperature is reached then place chicken in the air fryer basket.

Turn chicken halfway through. Serve and enjoy.

Chicken Burgers

Preparation Time: 10 minutes

Cooking Time: 18 minutes

Serve: 4

Ingredients:

1 lb ground chicken

3 oz almond flour

1 tbsp oregano

2 oz mozzarella cheese, shredded

Pepper

Salt

Directions:

Add all ingredients into the mixing bowl and mix until well combined.

Make 4 equal shapes of patties from meat mixture.

Select Air Fry mode.

Set time to 18 minutes and temperature 360 F then press START.

The air fryer display will prompt you to ADD FOOD once the temperature is reached then place chicken patties in the air fryer basket.

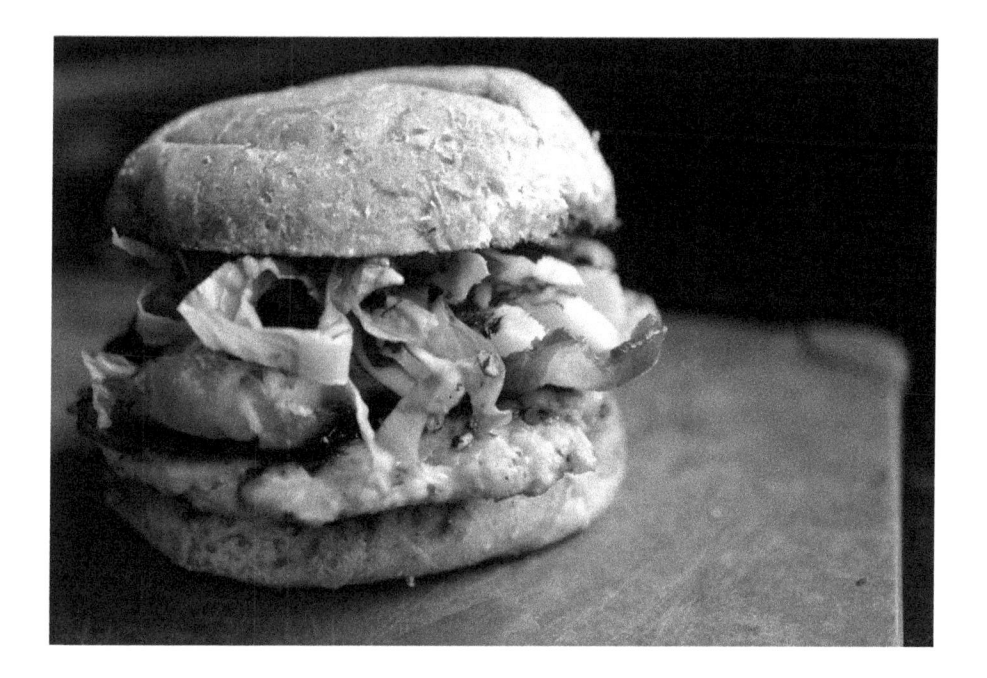

Serve and enjoy

Tasty Chicken Tenders

Preparation Time: 10 minutes

Cooking Time: 16 minutes

Serve: 4

Ingredients:

1 lb chicken tenders

For rub:

1/2 tbsp dried thyme

1 tbsp garlic powder

1 tbsp paprika

1/2 tbsp onion powder

1/2 tsp cayenne pepper

Pepper

Salt

Directions:

In a bowl, add all rub ingredients and mix well.

Add chicken tenders into the bowl and coat with rub.

Select Air Fry mode.

Set time to 16 minutes and temperature 370 F then press START.

The air fryer display will prompt you to ADD FOOD once the temperature is reached then place chicken tenders in the air fryer basket.

Turn chicken tenders halfway through.

Jerk Chicken

Preparation Time: 10 minutes

Cooking Time: 20 minutes

Serve: 2

Ingredients:

1 lb chicken wings

1 tbsp jerk seasoning

1 tsp olive oil

Pepper

Salt

Directions:

In a mixing bowl, add chicken wings.

Add remaining ingredients on top of chicken wings and toss to coat.

Select Air Fry mode.

Set time to 20 minutes and temperature 380 F then press START.

The air fryer display will prompt you to ADD FOOD once the temperature is reached then place chicken wings in the air fryer basket.

Serve and enjoy.

Chicken Fritters

Preparation Time: 10 minutes

Cooking Time: 25 minutes

Serve: 4

Ingredients:

1 lb ground chicken

1 1/2 cups mozzarella cheese, shredded

1/2 cup onion, chopped

2 cups broccoli, chopped

3/4 cup almond flour

2 garlic cloves, minced

1 egg, lightly beaten

Pepper

Salt

Directions:

Add all ingredients into the mixing bowl and mix until well combined.

Make small patties from the meat mixture.

Select Bake mode.

Set time to 25 minutes and temperature 380 F then press START.

The air fryer display will prompt you to ADD FOOD once the temperature is reached then place chicken patties in the air fryer basket.

Turn patties halfway through.

Serve and enjoy.

Chicken Nuggets

Preparation Time: 10 minutes

Cooking Time: 25 minutes

Serve: 4

Ingredients:

1 1/2 lbs chicken breast, boneless & cut into chunks

1/2 tsp garlic powder

1/4 cup parmesan cheese, shredded

1/4 cup mayonnaise

1/4 tsp salt

Directions:

In a bowl, mix together mayonnaise, cheese, garlic powder, and salt.

Add chicken and mix until well coated.

Select Air Fry mode.

Set time to 25 minutes and temperature 400 F then press START.

The air fryer display will prompt you to ADD FOOD once the temperature is reached then add chicken in the air fryer basket.

Serve and enjoy

Garlic Butter Wings

Preparation Time: 10 minutes

Cooking Time: 25 minutes

Serve: 3

Ingredients:

1 lb chicken wings

1/2 tsp Italian seasoning

1 tsp garlic powder

1/4 tsp pepper

1/2 tsp salt

For sauce:

1 tbsp butter, melted

1/8 tsp garlic powder

Directions:

In a bowl, toss chicken wings with Italian seasoning, garlic powder, pepper, and salt.

Select Air Fry mode.

Set time to 25 minutes and temperature 390 F then press START.

The air fryer display will prompt you to ADD FOOD once the temperature is reached then add chicken wings in the air fryer basket.

In a large bowl, mix together melted butter and garlic powder.

Add chicken wings and toss until well coated. Serve and enjoy.

Jalapeno Meatballs

Preparation Time: 10 minutes

Cooking Time: 25 minutes

Serve: 4

Ingredients:

1 lb ground chicken

1/2 cup cilantro, chopped

1 jalapeno pepper, minced

1 habanero pepper, minced

1 poblano chili pepper, minced

Salt

Directions:

Add all ingredients into the large bowl and mix until well combined.

Make small balls from the meat mixture.

Select Air Fry mode.

Set time to 25 minutes and temperature 400 F then press START.

The air fryer display will prompt you to ADD FOOD once the temperature is reached then place meatballs in the air fryer basket.

Serve and enjoy

Thyme Sage Turkey

Breast Preparation Time: 10 minutes

Cooking Time: 60 minutes

Serve: 8

Ingredients:

1 lbs turkey breast

1/4 tsp pepper

1 tbsp butter

1/2 tsp sage leaves, chopped

1/2 tsp thyme leaves, chopped

1 tsp salt

Directions:

Rub butter all over the turkey breast and season with pepper, sage, thyme, and salt.

Select Bake mode.

Set time to 60 minutes and temperature 325 F then press START.

The air fryer display will prompt you to ADD FOOD once the temperature is reached then place turkey breast in the air fryer basket.

Turn turkey breast halfway through.

Serve and enjoy.

Flavorful Spiced Chicken

Preparation Time: 10 minutes

Cooking Time: 10 minutes

Serve: 8

Ingredients:

2 lbs chicken thigh, skinless and boneless

1/2 tsp ground ginger

1 tbsp cayenne

1 tbsp cinnamon

1 tbsp coriander powder

3 tbsp coconut oil, melted

1/2 tsp ground nutmeg

Pepper

Salt

Directions:

In a small bowl, mix together all spices.

Brush chicken with oil and rub with spice mixture.

Season with salt.

Select Air Fry mode.

Set time to 10 minutes and temperature 390 F then press START.

The air fryer display will prompt you to ADD FOOD once the temperature is reached then place chicken in the air fryer basket.

Serve and enjoy.

Persian Kabab

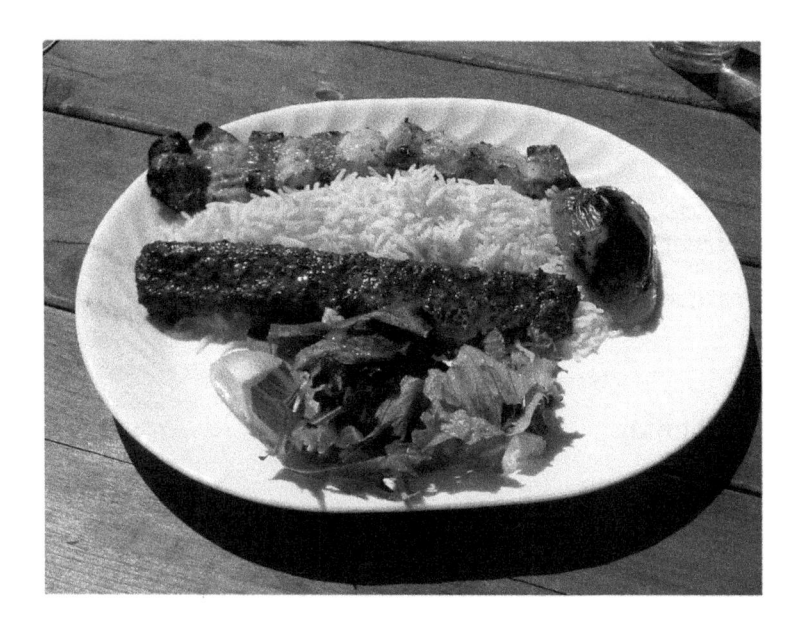

Preparation Time: 10 minutes

Cooking Time: 6 minutes

Serve: 3

Ingredients:

1 lb ground chicken

1/4 cup almond flour

2 green onion, chopped

1 egg, lightly beaten

1/3 cup fresh parsley, chopped

2 garlic cloves

4 oz onion, chopped

1/4 tsp turmeric powder

1/2 tsp black pepper

1 tbsp fresh lemon juice

Directions:

Add all ingredients into the food processor and process until well combined.

Transfer chicken mixture to the bowl and place it in the refrigerator for 30 minutes.

Divide mixture into the six equal portions and roll around the soaked wooden skewers.

Select Air Fry mode.

Set time to 6 minutes and temperature 400 F then press START.

The air fryer display will prompt you to ADD FOOD once the temperature is reached then place chicken skewers in the air fryer basket.

Serve and enjoy.

Asian Chicken Wings

Preparation Time: 10 minutes

Cooking Time: 30 minutes

Serve: 2

Ingredients:

4 chicken wings

1 tbsp soy sauce

1 tbsp Chinese spice

1 tsp mixed spice

Pepper

Salt

Directions:

Add chicken wings into the bowl.

Add remaining ingredients and toss well.

Select Air Fry mode.

Set time to 30 minutes and temperature 350 F then press START.

The air fryer display will prompt you to ADD FOOD once the temperature is reached then place chicken wings in the air fryer basket.

Turn chicken wings halfway through.

Spicy Chicken Wings

Preparation Time: 10 minutes

Cooking Time: 25 minutes

Serve: 4

Ingredients:

2 lbs chicken wings

6 tbsp butter, melted

12 oz hot sauce

1 tsp chili powder

Directions:

Select Air Fry mode.

Set time to 25 minutes and temperature 380 F then press START.

The air fryer display will prompt you to ADD FOOD once the temperature is reached then place chicken wings in the air fryer basket.

Meanwhile, in a bowl, mix together hot sauce, butter, and chili powder.

Add cooked chicken wings into the sauce bowl and toss well.

Serve and enjoy.

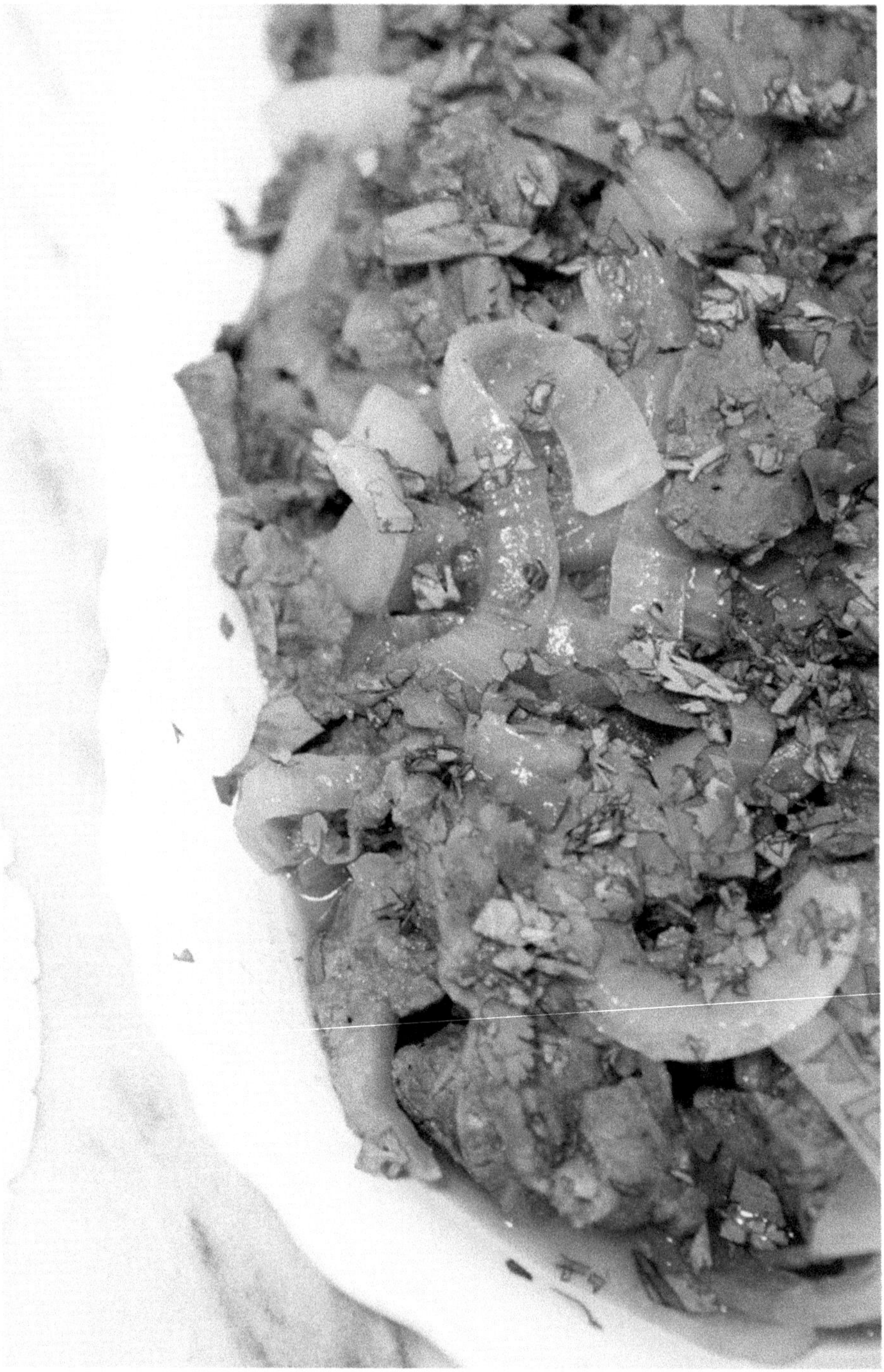